Amelia Woods
P.O. Box 11451
Pensacola, FL 32524

www.heartlikeamother.com

ISBN 979-8-9879719-6-3 hardcover
ISBN 979-8-9879719-7-0 paperback

Library of Congress Control Number: 2024902206

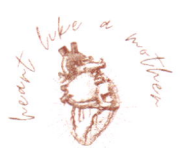
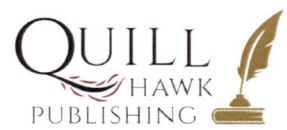

This book is dedicated to you, Henderson Jude. May you always "take a sad song and make it better".
Love, Mom

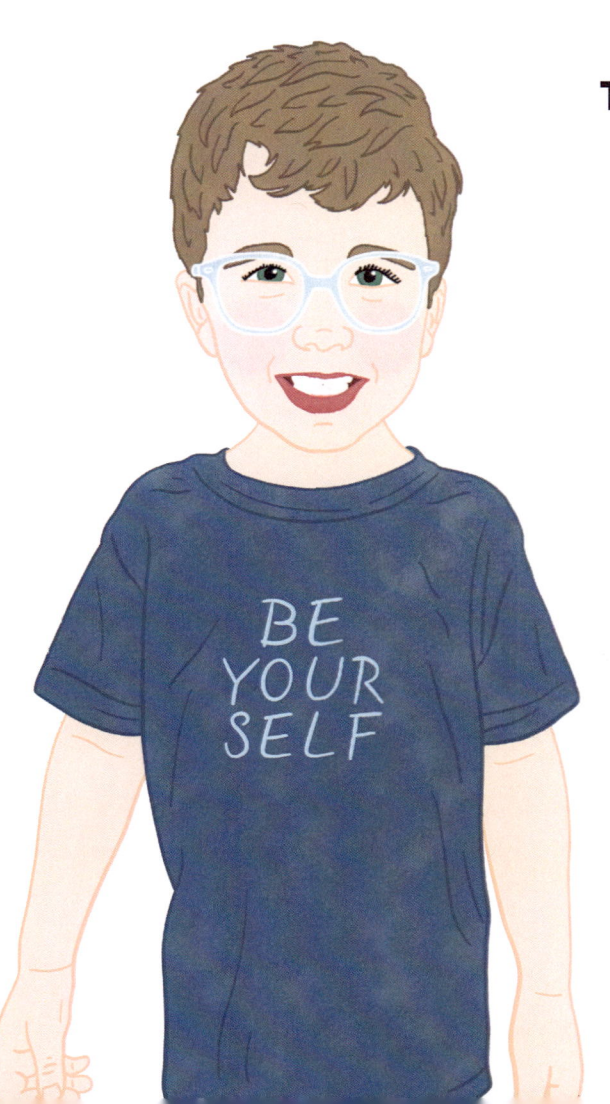

My heart is special, yes, it's true!
This book is a letter from me to you.

When I was a baby, my heart
needed fixing. So, doctors
worked hard to fix what
needed switching.

You see, I was born with an extra special heart,

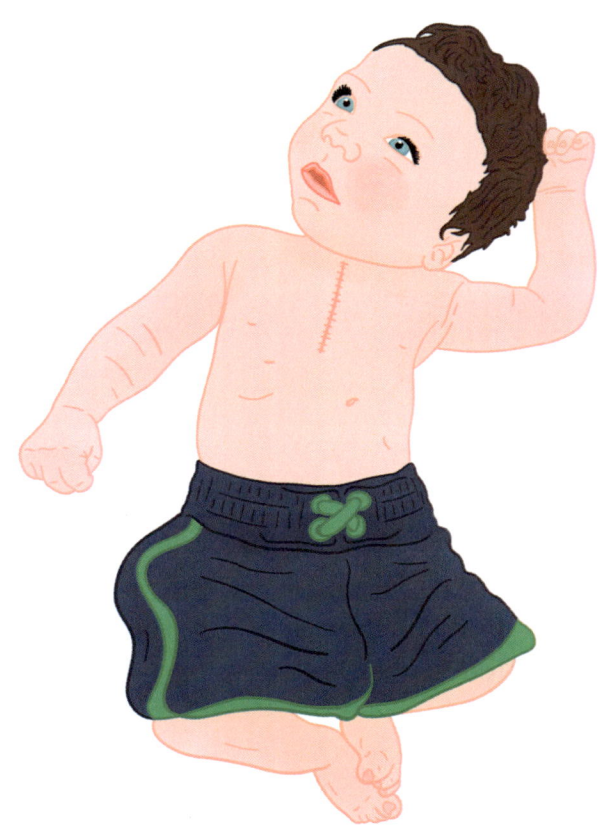

my family tells me I've been brave from the start!

In my special heart, parts needed
swapping to help it beat strong

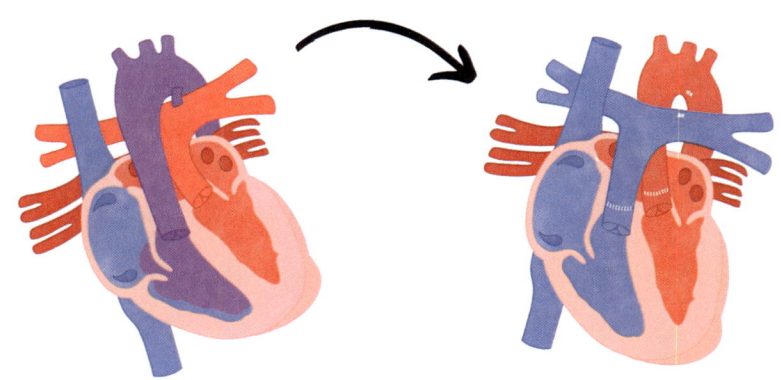

so I was given a
whole team to help
me along!

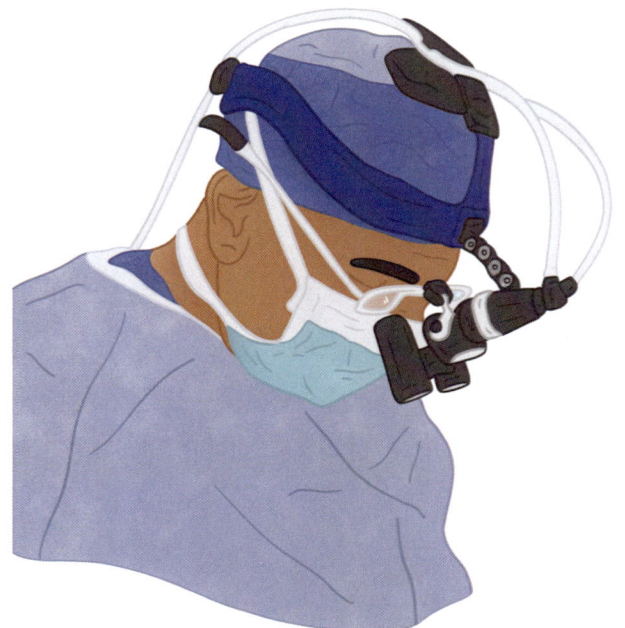

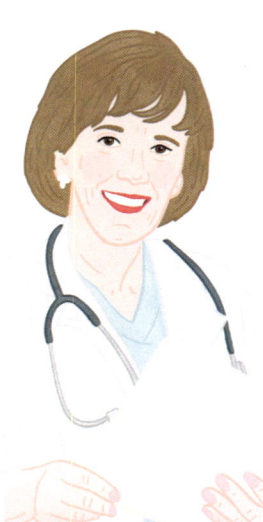

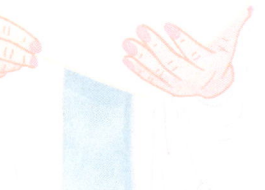

The doctors, the nurses, and therapists who cared for me, made sure I stayed well and helped ease my family's worries.

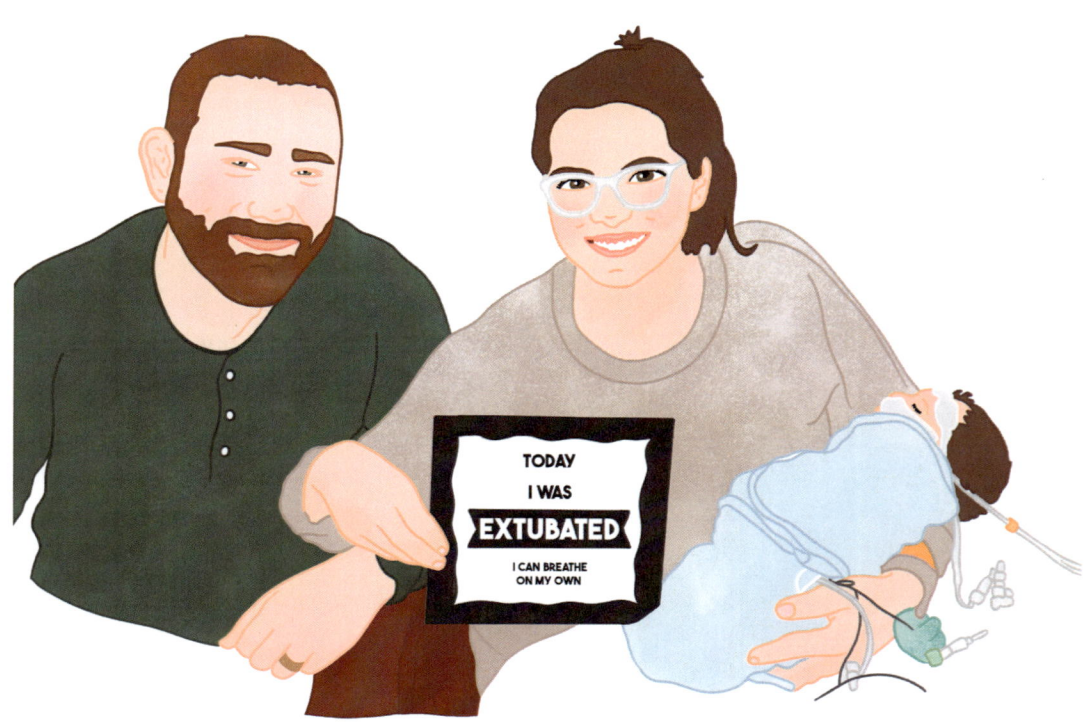

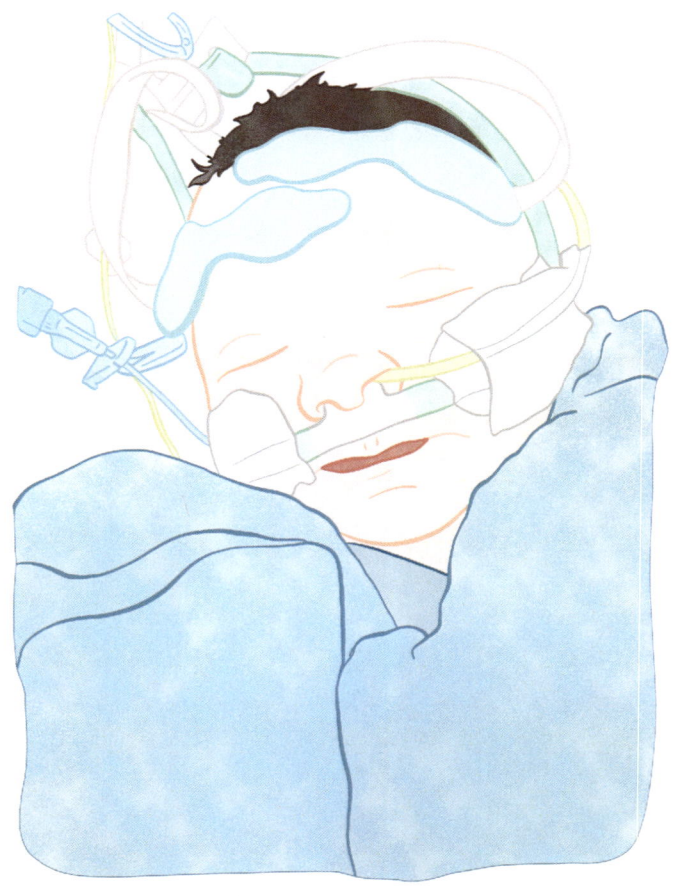

I spent lots of time in the hospital, longer than most babies do.

But that's because my special team had
important work to get through!

God's hands led the way to fix my special heart, He gives cardiologists and surgeons the tools for their art.

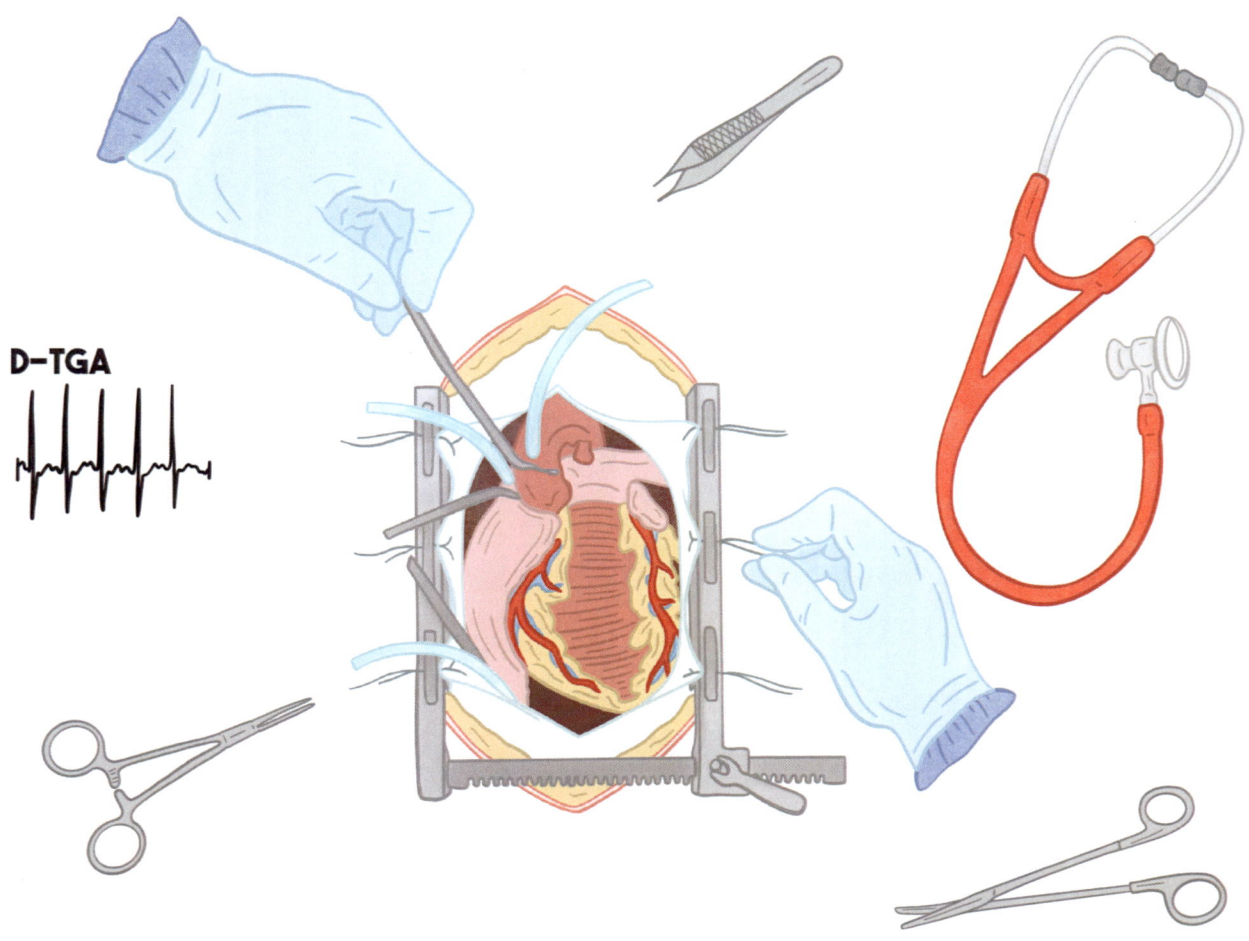

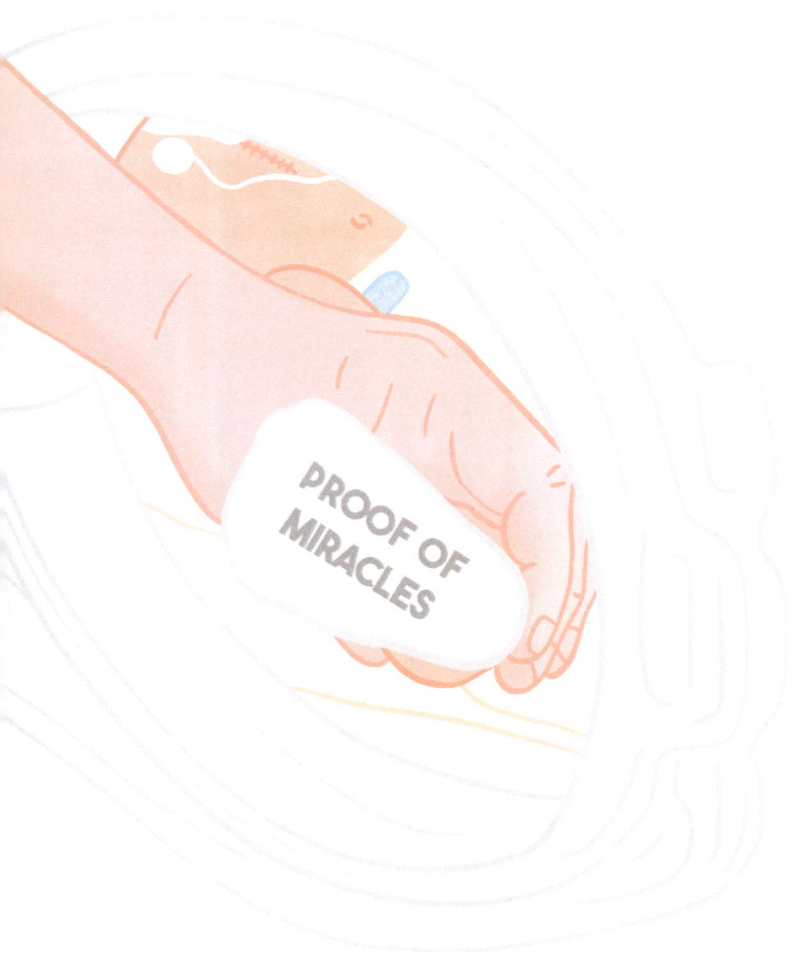

When I look at my scar, I know this to be true: special hearts come from God, who created me and you!

When I look at my scar, I feel big and strong!

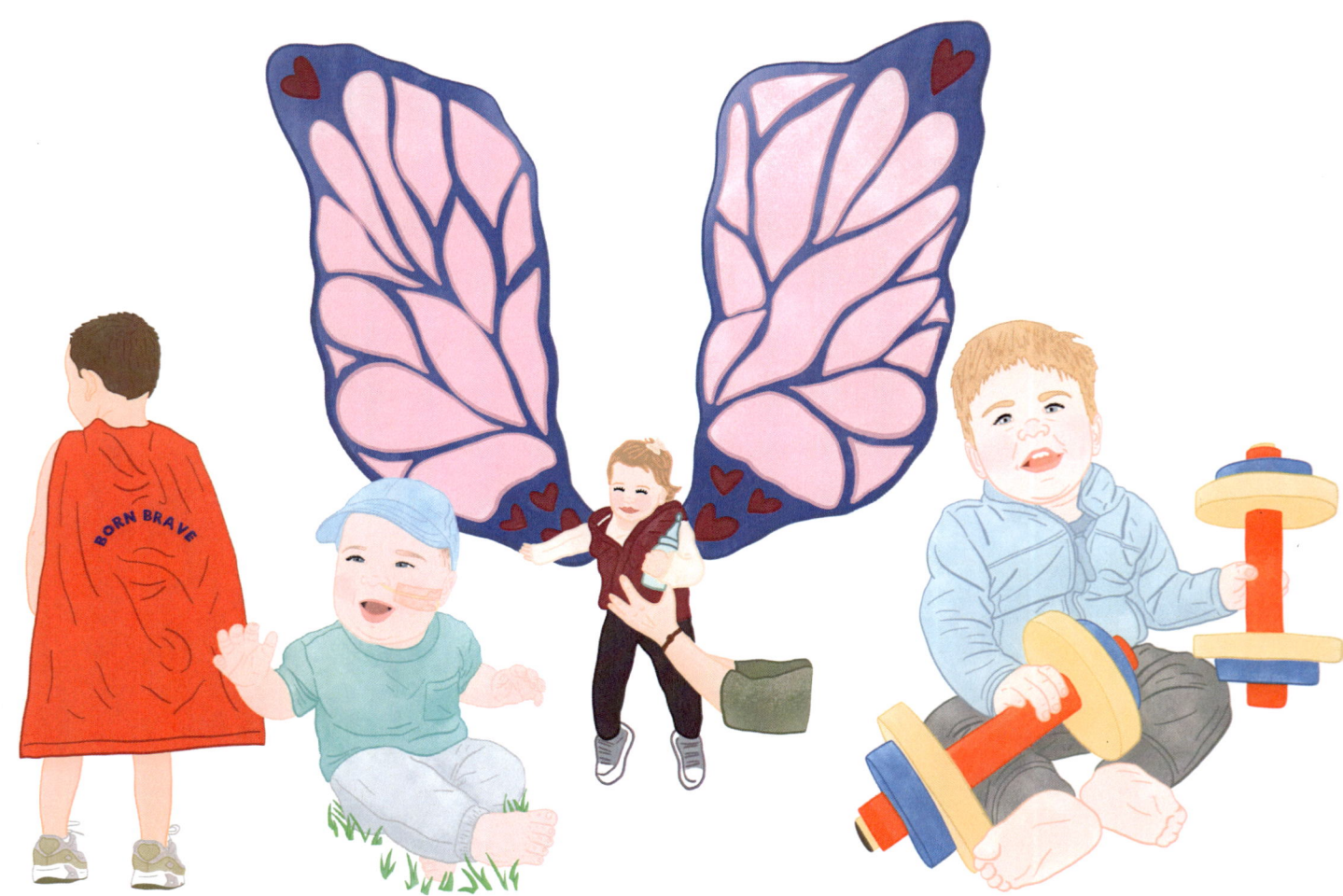

I know anything is possible for me, and that I've been brave all along.

When I look at my scar,
I am reminded of life's
blessings.

I know I have a purpose, in that
there's no guessing!

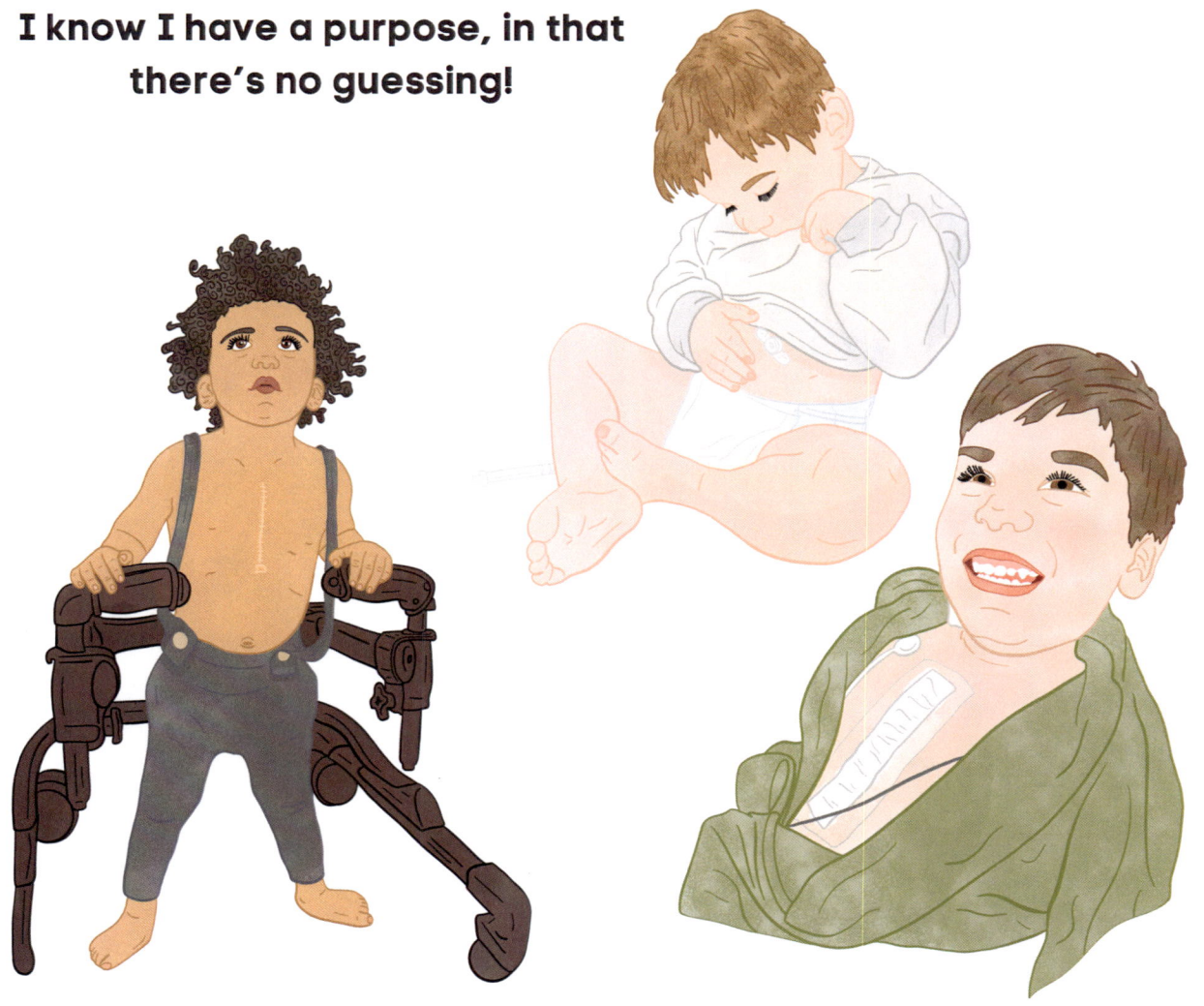

Having a special heart does not hold me back,
it's just part of my life's story,
it's as simple as that!

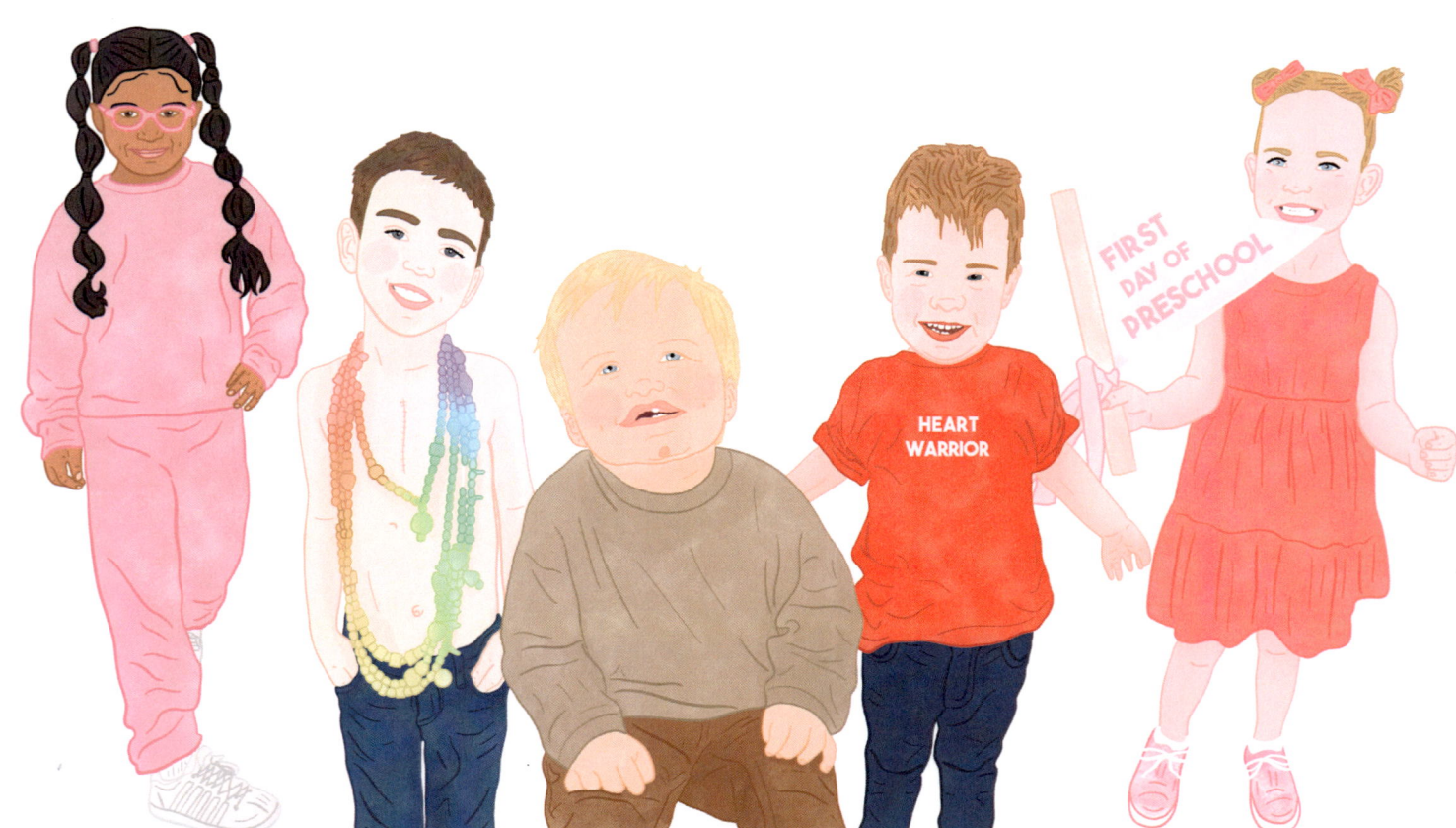

If you have a heart like mine, remind yourself of these things:

You wear a symbol of your bravery
and it is unique to you.

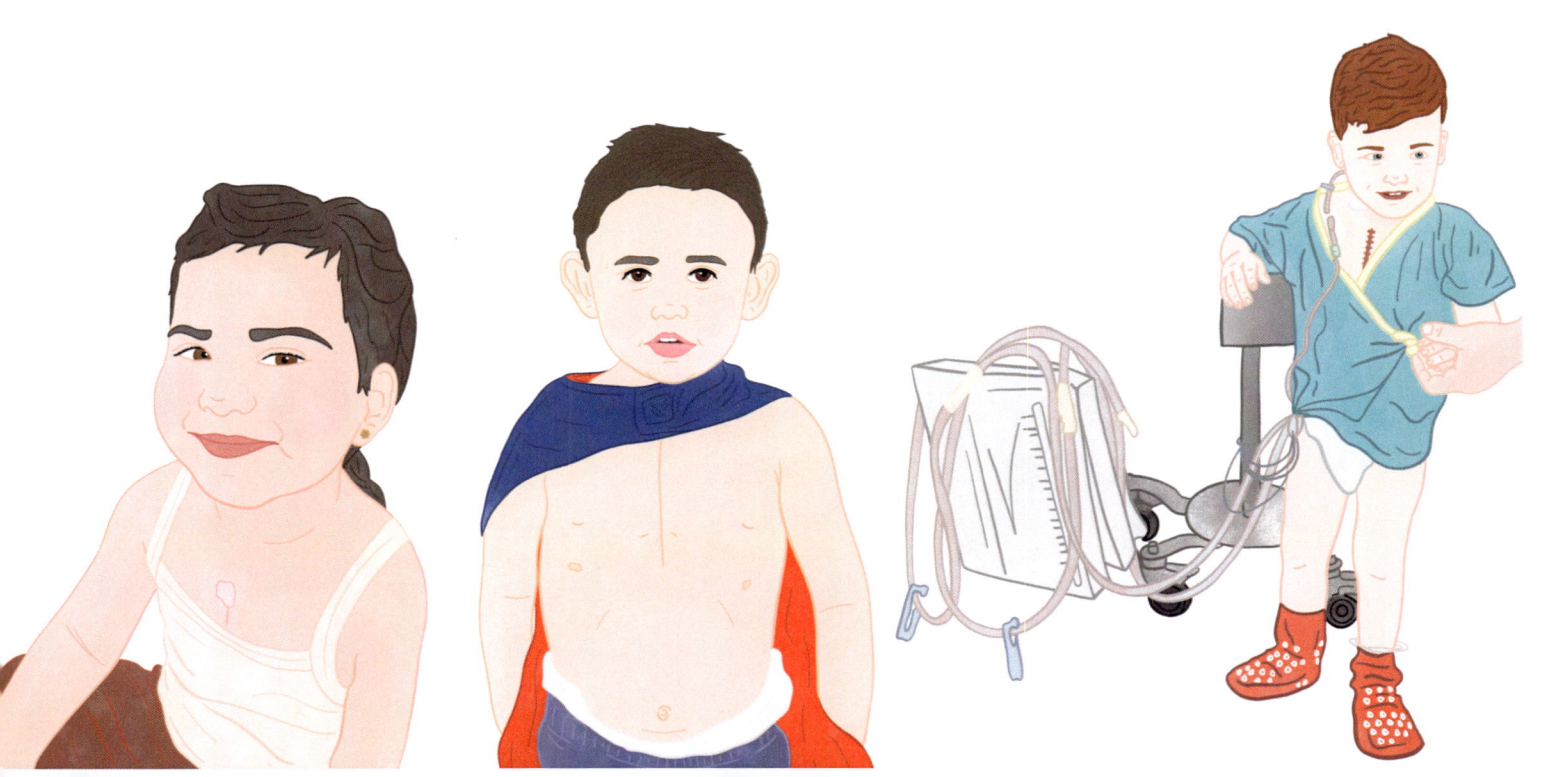

Your scar is a line that shows all
you can do.

You can play,
you can dream,
even be part of a team!

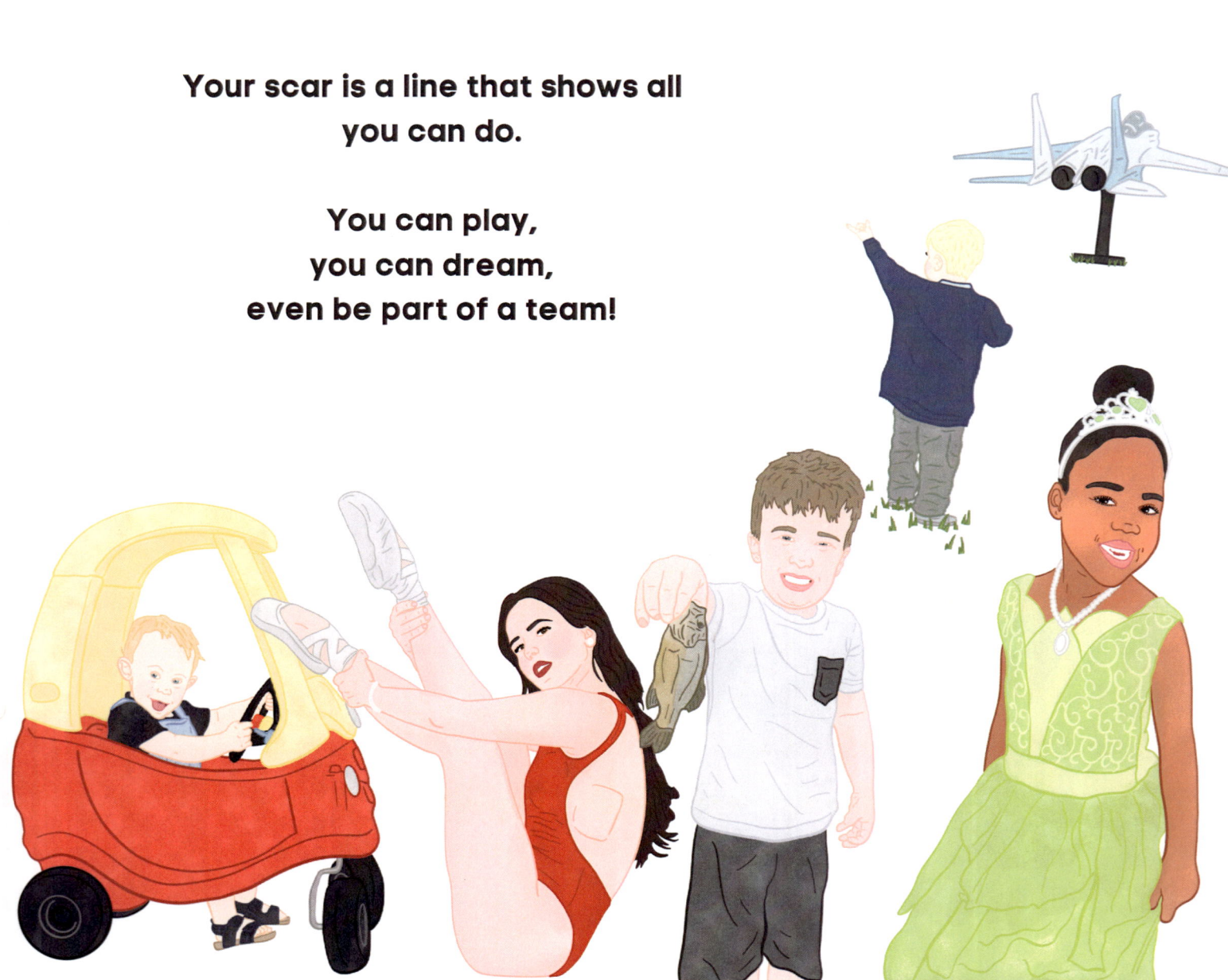

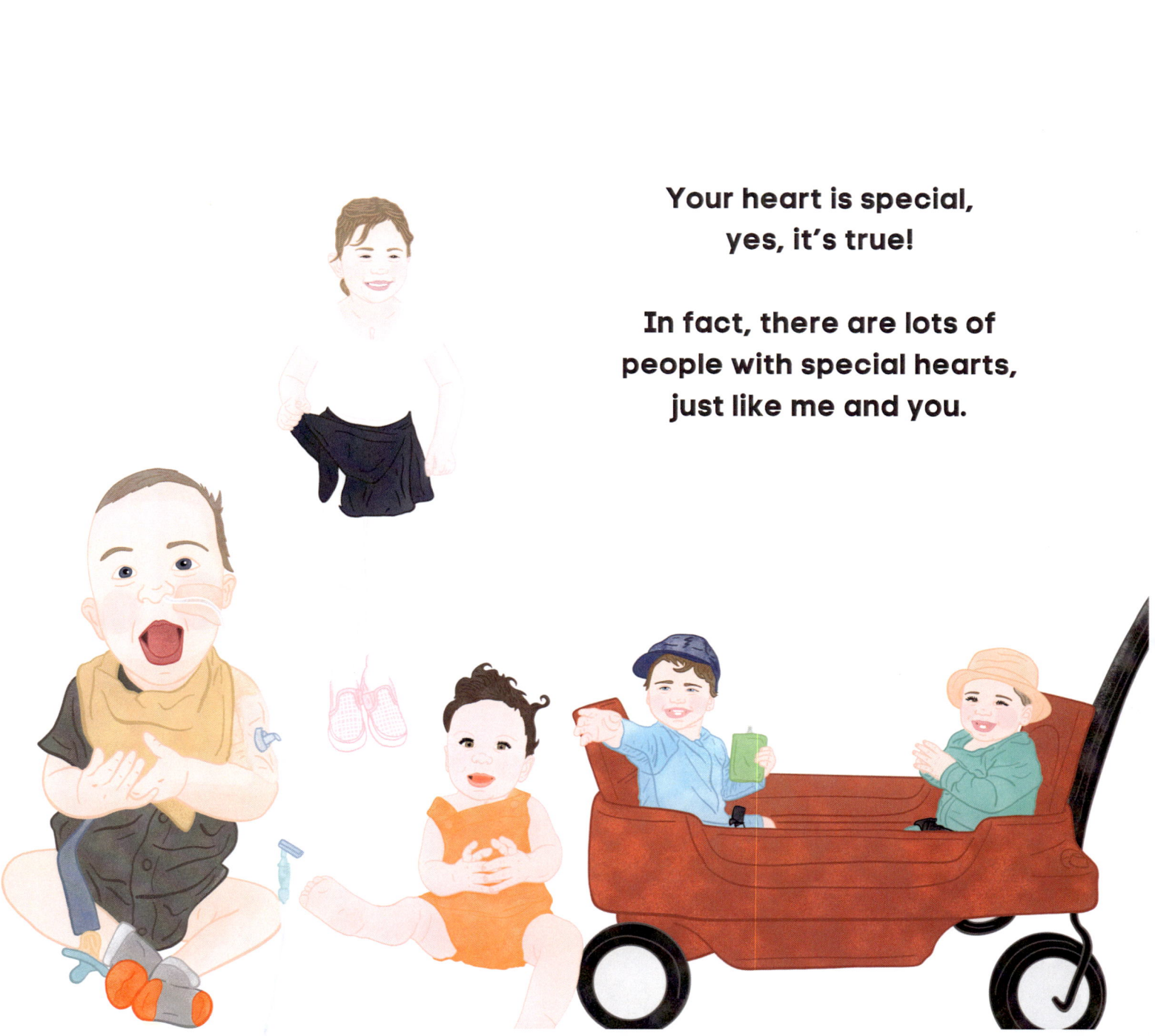

Your heart is special,
yes, it's true!

In fact, there are lots of
people with special hearts,
just like me and you.

Being born brave means you were tough from the start.

Since day one, we've fought battles with our extra special hearts.

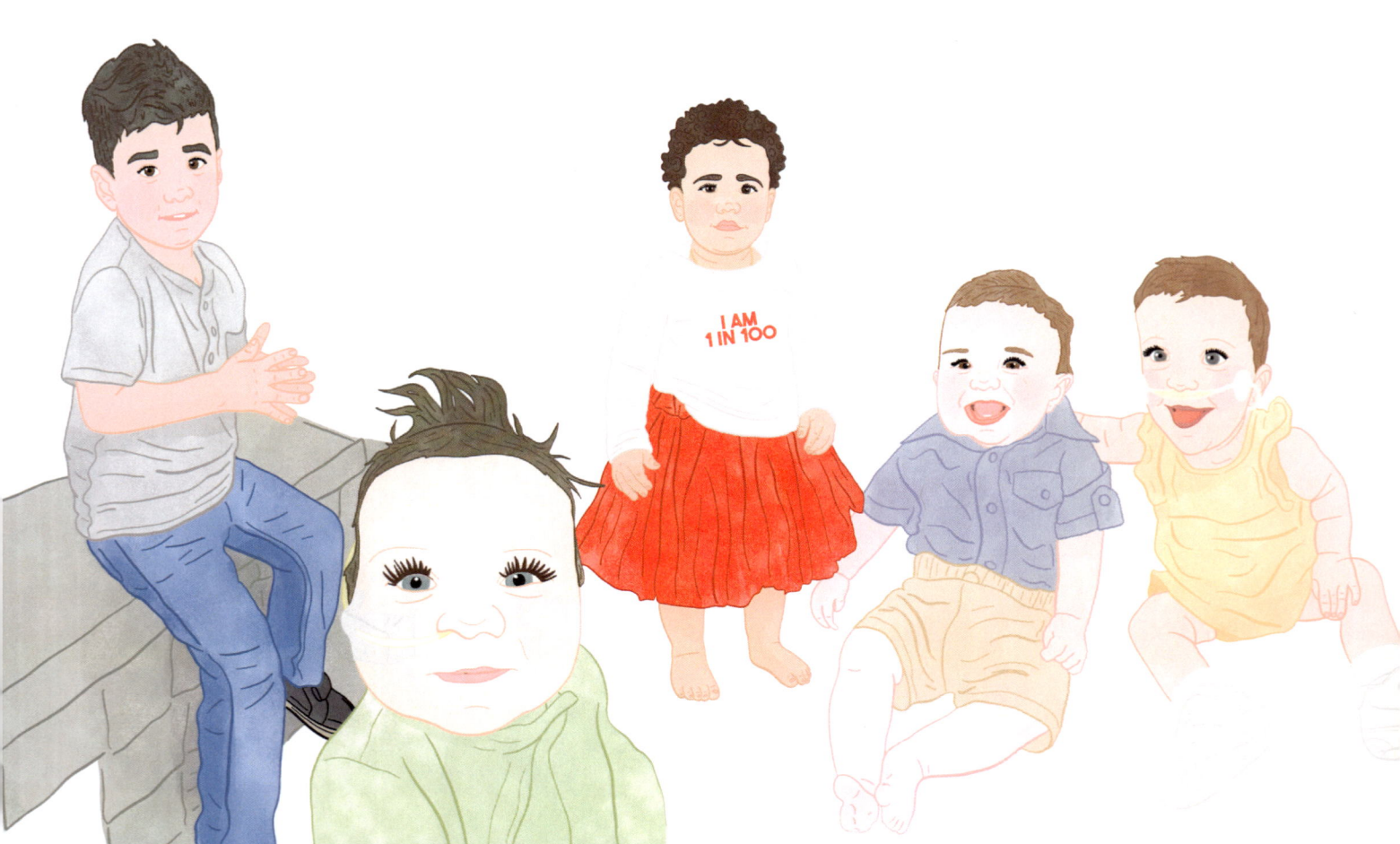

Now, your heart might beat normal, and that is special, too.

Your heart is built to beat the best it can for you!

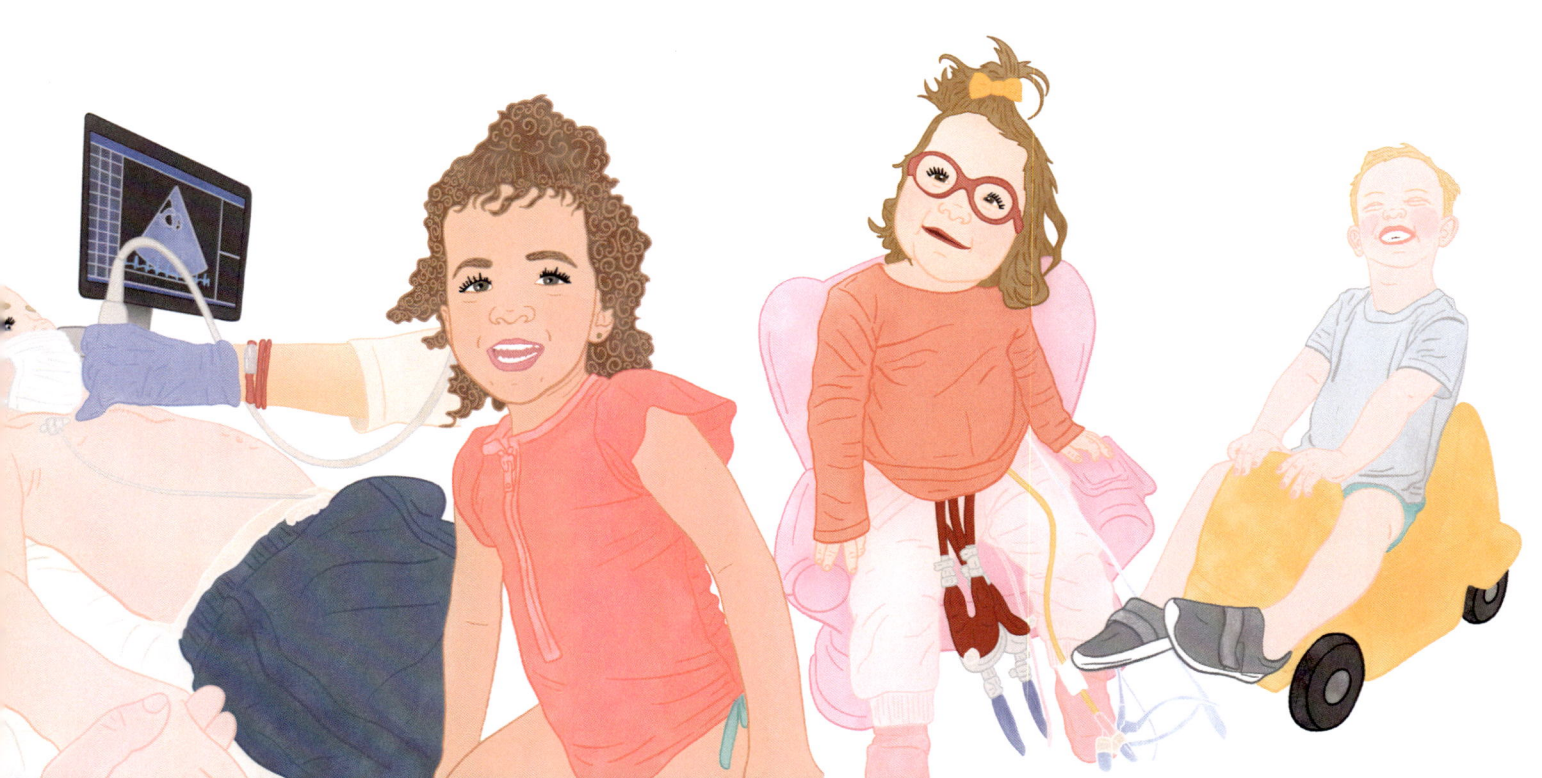

Whether you're like me or not, no one's heart is the same.

It's important to remember being different is okay.

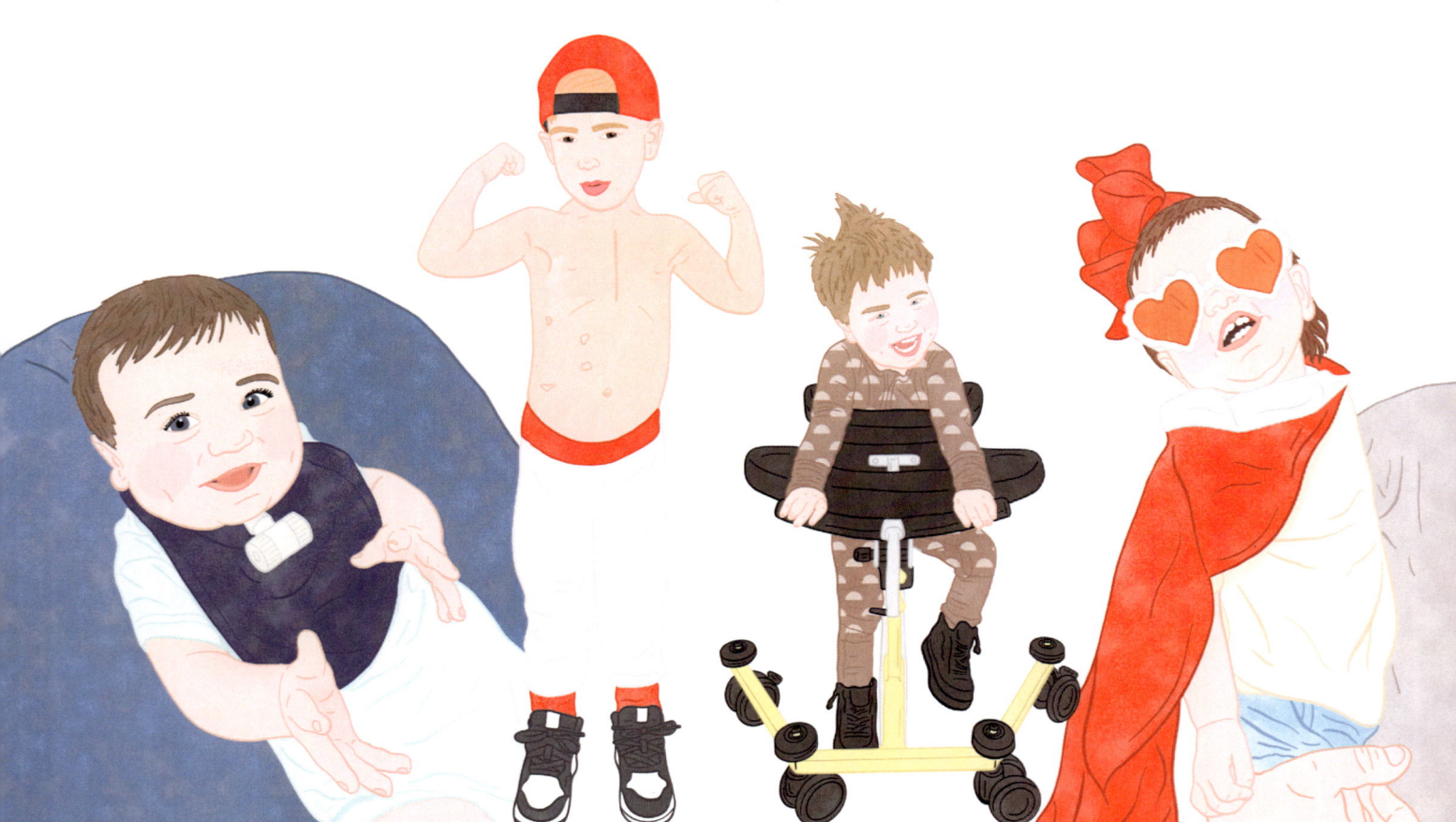

About the Author
Amelia Woods

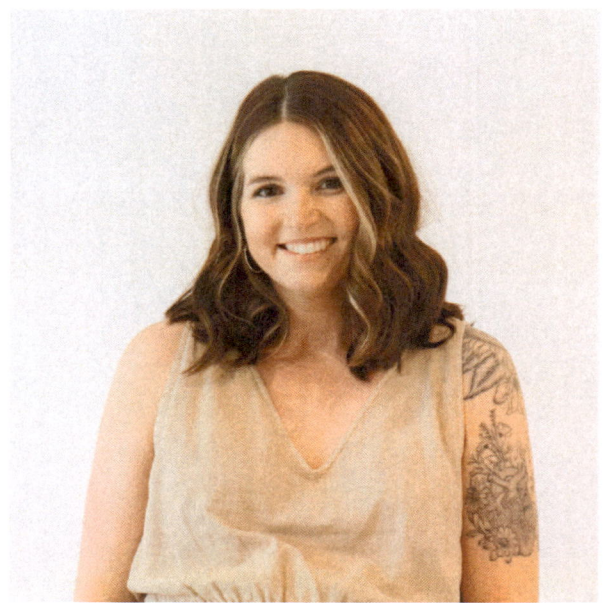

Amelia was born and raised in Pensacola, Florida and lives there today with her two boys and husband. Her unique journey into motherhood began with her oldest son's CHD diagnosis of d-TGA, which inspired her to create the blog and online platform Heart Like A Mother. She is driven to support other parents of children with Congenital Heart Disease in any way possible. Her hope in writing The Boy Born Brave is that it highlights the diversity within the CHD community, brings encouragement to new parents facing a diagnosis for their child, and educates those of us with "normal" hearts.

About the Illustrator
Hannah Conrad

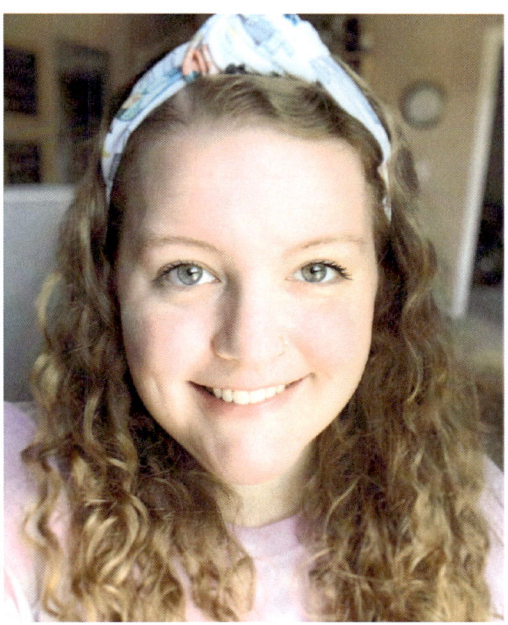

Hannah is a digital artist and creator whose passion is to raise awareness for CHD and provide representation for medical families! Through her journey with her very own heart warrior she's found outlets for giving back to others on their own heart and medical journeys by serving on the board for Sisters by Heart, her small business Studio142, and serving as programs coordinator for The Healing Hearts Project. When not busy with all these fun things you can either catch her with her nose in a book or chasing her kids around the nearest park.

Special Thanks from The Author

While this story was written with my own child in mind, I can honestly say that the execution of this project could not have happened without the support of all those I've come to know in the Congenital Heart community. To all the parents of CHD warriors, and to the Adult CHD warriors who have shared their stories and experiences with me, thank you. To the families of heart angels, thank you for continuing to share your loved one's light with the world even in the midst of your grief; I know they are proud of you for showing up for them. To the families of warriors pictured throughout this book, thank you for allowing me to include a piece of you in the pages of this story. I am forever grateful to you, my fellow CHD parents, for sharing your perspectives, experiences, advice, support, and most of all, friendship.

May you all know just how BRAVE you have been from the start!

Amelia ♡